Who's Afraid?

WHO'S AFRAID?
The Phobic's Handbook

by Barbara Fried

Illustrated by Robert Seaver, M.D.

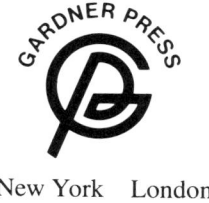

New York   London

Who's Afraid?

Copyright © 1985 by Barbara Fried
All rights reserved.
No part of this book may be reproduced
in any form,
by photostat, microform, retrieval system,
or any means now known or later devised,
without prior written permission of the publisher.

Reprinted with new illustrations from 1971 edition by McGraw-Hill.

Gardner Press, Inc.
19 Union Square West
New York 10003

All foreign orders except Canada and South America to:
Afterhurst Limited
Chancery House
319 City Road
London N1, United Kingdom

Library of Congress Cataloging in Publication Data

Fried, Barbara.
  Who's afraid?

  Originally published: New York: McGraw-Hill, 1971.
  1. Phobias. I. Title.
RC535.F75   1985   616.85'225   84-28671
ISBN 0-89876-104-2

PRINTED IN THE UNITED STATES OF AMERICA

for Richard the Lion-Hearted

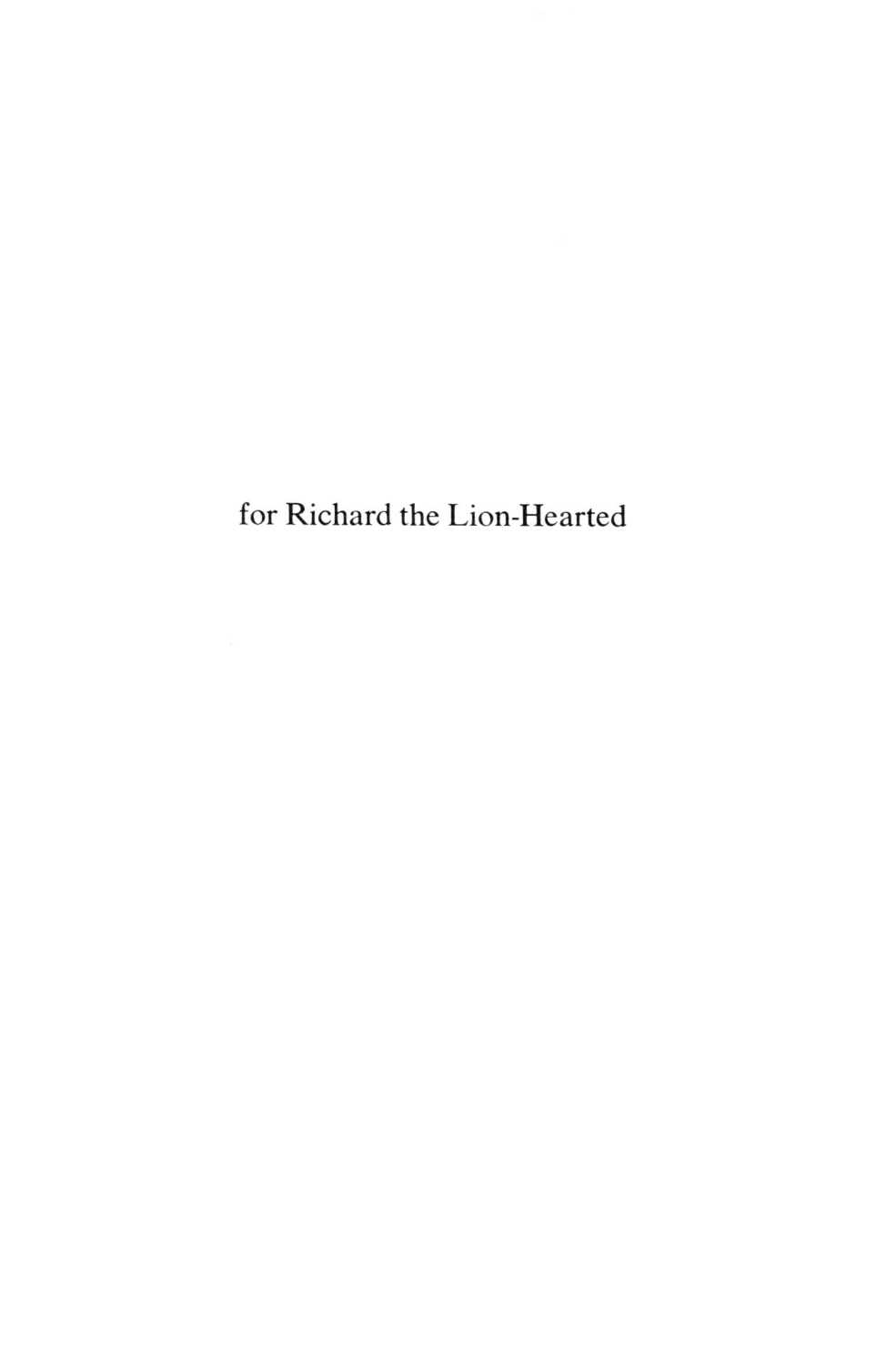

Who's Afraid?

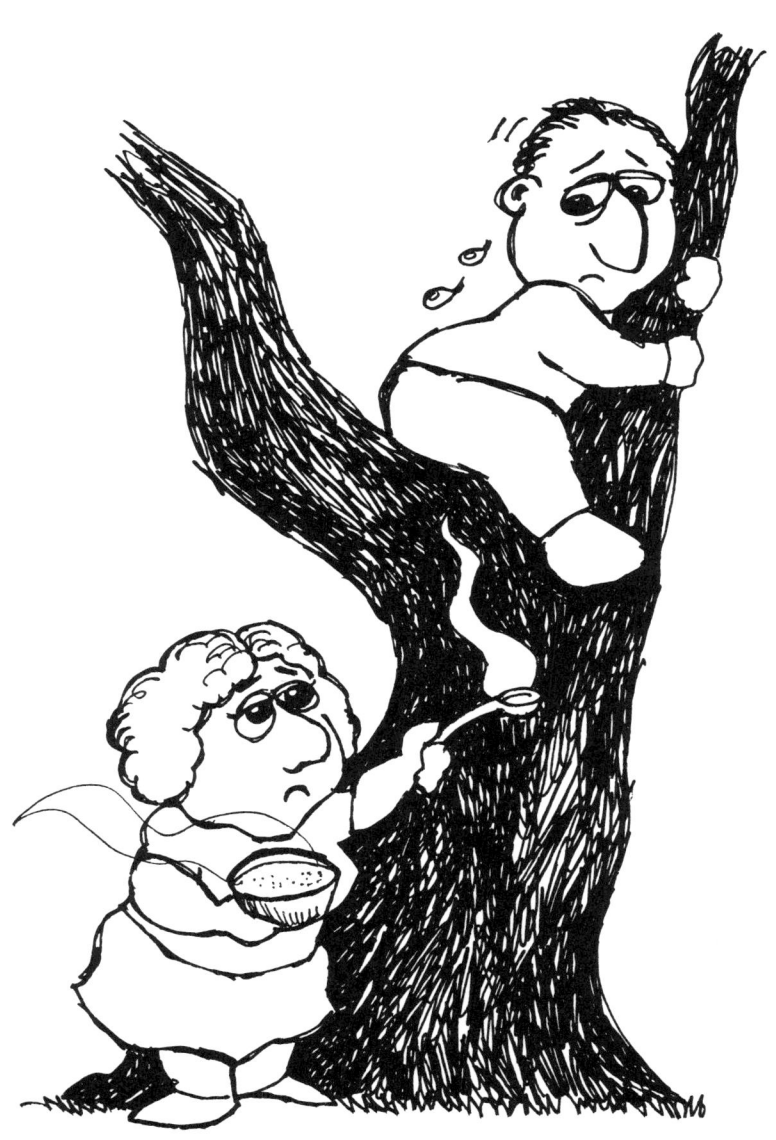

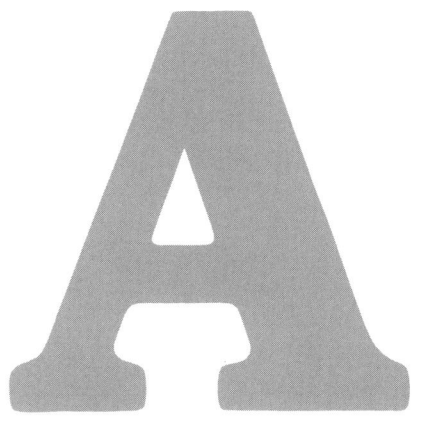

*A is for Anxiety
From transient to acute.
Phobia's one variety
And, man, it is a beaut!*

ANXIETY

A phobia is an intense and irrationally fearful anxiety—a morbid dread—provoked by some object, situation, or idea that is not actually harmful. Here are a few of the physical and mental symptoms that may occur when a phobic has to face, see, or think about what terrifies him: extreme restlessness, rapid heart rate, palpitations, pains anywhere in the body, numbness, nausea, vomiting, diarrhea, weakness,

A

dizziness, fainting, instant fatigue, inability to concentrate or remember, and an overwhelming urge to go elsewhere immediately, if not sooner. There are others, all just as bad. It is obvious that for symptoms like these, chicken soup won't even come close.

You may think these panic reactions are happening to you because you're afraid of the phobic object, idea, or situation itself. That's all you know. According to psychoanalytic theory, the phobic object is only a symbolic representation of an internal conflict (*see also* Association, Displacement, and Symbol). Unconsciously you're really anxious about something else entirely,* and the phobia merely serves as its substitute in the real world.

You may or may not go along with this analytic point of view.** But the hypothesis that a phobic situation, object, or idea is actually a dream desire in dread disguise is supported by two pieces of evidence: the characteristically irrational nature of phobias in general, and the fantastic intensity of the anxiety you feel when you confront your own special phobic thing.

It's true that in a world where television sets radiate silent menace in a corner of your living room, and where the very air you breathe is killing you, the line between what is and what is not realistically dangerous does tend to be rather fuzzy. Nonetheless, everyone will probably agree that caterpillars, cats, thunder, a bowl of fruit, blood, going over a

---

*What else, exactly, psychoanalytic theory is not sure, but the smart medical money seems to favor the notion that the unconscious anxiety is aroused by a combination of two things: (1) a temptation to gratify an instinctual sexual or aggressive desire—making it with your mother, say —and (2) a guilty fear of being punished if you go ahead and do it the way you really would like to. In other words, the thing a person is consciously phobic to symbolizes something he unconsciously wants. Stranger things have turned out to be true.

**There's no reason why you should. After all, not too long ago the smart medical money was betting that phobias were caused by an excess of black bile. *See also* Behaviorists.

12

A

bridge, the dark, automobile tailpipes, going to school, and butterflies are not in themselves harmful; yet all these things terrify somebody. A phobic will even admit that large shiny green leaves cannot possibly hurt him. After admitting it, however, he will go right on being afraid. And the more you try to talk him out of it, the quicker you make him go elsewhere.

Furthermore, even assuming his phobia involves something that is hazardous enough to make nonphobics nervous —flying, say—the phobic's anxiety is far greater than normal and out of all reasonable proportion to the actual risk.

Such totally unrealistic behavior can only mean that the phobic is not reacting to the object itself but that, instead, the object must stand for something else, although only to him—and that something else is what he's responding to. Which is to say that a phobic object, idea, or situation is actually a projection of an anxiety-provoking idea that your conscious mind doesn't want to know about, but that your unconscious mind insists on thinking about anyway.

The trouble is that the unconscious doesn't know from being reasonable, and the damn thing *never* forgets.

ACROPHOBIA

A morbid dread of heights or high places—bridges, roofs, tops or sides of mountains, Denver, glass-enclosed outside elevators, or even the seat of a chair when you have to climb up on it to change a light bulb. A common, nongarden phobia. Not the same as fear of flying—which, according to the people who have that, is really something else (*see* Claustrophobia). Freud remarked that people with acrophobia were

A

unconsciously afraid of becoming famous.* Other analysts have related acrophobia to an unconscious fear of detumescence. Logically those men who worry that their talent for detumescence will make them famous (or at least notorious) among their friends ought to suffer from double acrophobia —but of course they don't, because phobias aren't logical.

Acrophobia very neatly shows how a phobia simultaneously represents in the real world both aspects of an unconscious conflict—both a desire for some forbidden thing and a fear of being punished for trying to get it. On a conscious level we all are aware that heights symbolize success, fame, fortune, your name in lights, or, to put it succinctly, victory! We are all urged daily to achieve the pinnacle of success and to climb every mountain. On an unconscious level, too, you naturally want to be aggressive and win, so that you can be the top. That's one part of the unconscious conflict. The other part is that winning means to your unconscious that you conquer and kill, which as far as your superego (conscience) is concerned is definitely a no-no.

Back in the real world, then, the high place you're afraid of symbolizes an unconscious temptation to succeed; and that terrible feeling you get in the back of your knees that makes you sure you're going to fall and/or jump off when you look down represents the punishment being imposed by your conscience for wanting to kill—namely, to kill yourself. Someone who is really hung up on this conflict can barely manage to stand on tiptoe and is generally a failure in practically anything he tries to do.

On an everyday level, acrophobia tends to be an extremely inconvenient anxiety, especially for a city-dweller. Life being what it is these days, sooner or later everybody has to go into one of those all-glass apartment or office buildings; if you're

---

*Freud himself *loved* being famous, but he seems to have had a little trouble getting onto a train.

an acrophobe, you may be better off to try to do your business by phone. Interior corridors, elevators, and inside offices may be no problem—if they are, as a phobic you'll surely find some excuse to avoid going at all—since as long as you can't see out you may not have to admit that you're actually off the ground. You cannot hide it from yourself, however, when you're ushered into an outside office and find yourself thirty-five stories up with nothing between you and midair but a transparent pane of brownish-pink glass. Many a severely acrophobic person in this situation has dropped to the floor screaming and crawled out of the room clutching the carpet.* This behavior is not conducive to making a good impression on strong-jawed executive types, but there it is.

Mildly acrophobic people may be able to survive in this kind of office building, on the other hand, providing that they move their desks around so that their backs are to the window and they can concentrate their entire attention on the nice solid floor and walls. A good excuse for doing this is to say that the light hurts your eyes.

The urban terrace is another modern invention that acrophobes could—and of course do—live without. Some may be able to venture a step or so out onto one, especially if they're dragged bodily by an idiotic host, but generally they aren't able to appreciate the so-called spectacular view anyway, since the white-knuckled hand that is not clawing for a hold on the brick wall is clamped tightly over their eyes.

---

*One agent for such an office building says that when he started to rent space he used to run across the room and throw himself against the window wall to show how safe it was. He stopped bothering when he noticed that most of his prospective tenants never stayed around long enough to watch him pick himself up. Furthermore, he got tired of bumping his head and getting nosebleeds.

A

ACTION THERAPY

Treatment that forces the phobic to confront and deal actively with what he fears. Action therapists tend to be bluff, hearty bullies who rise early, eat large healthy breakfasts, and generally spend their free time on weekends officiating at Little League games. They also smile a lot and are never overweight. If Teddy Roosevelt were alive today, he'd make a dandy action therapist.

AGORAPHOBIA

Morbid dread that has to do with some aspect of open space —especially crossing or being alone in the middle of an empty space, like a field or a wide road. The open space itself, particularly when it's a street, may represent the temptation to indulge in sexual adventures (which is, after all, what *streetwalker* means); or, because it is open, it may represent a place where you both see others and are yourself also seen doing something bad—what, only your unconscious knows.

Supposedly the conflict in some cases of agoraphobia lies between an intense desire to show off—to go out there and knock 'em dead—and strong fears of being punished for wanting to be so aggressive. An open space symbolizes both these unconscious ideas simultaneously, since it offers the phobic an empty stage to perform on and at the same time threatens him with an implied total lack of response to his

A

self-exhibition. A crowded place is no less of a problem. There is the ultimate temptation of a ready-made audience, but then the potential for aggression—for actually harming someone—is too much of a threat to face. Either way the agoraphobic reacts with panic in the streets.

For these and other reasons, severely agoraphobic people may find it difficult or even impossible to walk outside by themselves, to board a bus or train, cross a bridge when they come to it, or even go out of a familiar safe room alone. However, any or all of these activities may be possible as long as they have somebody with them to protect them both from themselves and from being punished. This companion must usually be somebody they know very well who plays, essentially, the role of a magical substitute parent.

Agoraphobia is very often associated with other psychiatric symptoms—generalized anxiety, depression, obsession—and is one of the most difficult phobias to treat, especially since few therapists (for whatever the reason) are willing to leave their offices to make house calls.

ANIMAL PHOBIAS

Animal phobias (see also Bird Phobias *and* Little Hans). This term refers to a morbid dread of animals—most usually birds, mice, cats, dogs, and snakes—and doesn't mean that the animals themselves are phobic, at least as far as we know. Most animal phobias develop before the age of five and disappear between the ages of nine and eleven. So if you're older than five and have never had an animal phobia, you're pretty safe. If you're younger than five, you have no business to be reading this book.

A

ASSOCIATION

Association (*see also* Displacement *and* Symbol). The sneaky way one thing mentally leads to another. To coin an aphorism, the road to phobic hell is paved with bad associations, since that's the way you pick which phobic object is going to symbolize your very own particular unconscious conflict.

Many associations are based on similarities of shape, size, and/or function. It is the most natural thing in the world to look at a firehose spraying water and be reminded of a man urinating, and does not mean at all that you have a dirty mind, because everybody else thinks of it too. These obvious associations are a part of everyone's mental vocabulary (although of course many of them are culturally rather than genetically determined), which accounts for the knowing winks and smiles that are inevitably directed at any woman foolish enough to admit in public that she's phobic to snakes. Associations to a phobic object may be influenced by socially conveyed relationships; but even when they are, they are always basically and entirely personal. You cannot understand what a phobic object means to anyone without knowing his individual history—and sometimes you can't understand it even then. We all know our own histories, and most of us don't have a clue about why we dread one thing rather than another.

A

AVOIDANCE

Avoidance (*see also* Counterphobia). The main psychic advantage of developing a phobia is that after you've displaced your unconscious anxiety onto a symbolic situation or object you are in a reasonably good position to avoid it. After all, practically any situation or object in the external real world is easier to get away from than something inside your own head.

You have to remember, though, that avoidance is not actually an attempt to escape from the phobic object itself, but from the anxiety you've transferred to it. That's why the desire to avoid has nothing to do with realistic danger; that's also why the need to avoid can be, and often is, unbelievably intense and totally uncontrollable. There are people who'd dive out a window before they'd spend two seconds in a room with an uncaged parakeet. And if you're between them and the window, they'd push you right out ahead of them if that's the only way they could get through. So watch out.

If our unconscious were only as sensible as it is devious, it would transfer its apprehension to some symbolic object it knew in advance we wouldn't be apt to run into very often in the course of a lifetime—an iceberg, say (well, all right, but how many other ships *besides* the *Titanic?*). Or a flying saucer. However, the unconscious is ludicrously shortsighted about most things, and as a result, since nobody likes feeling anxious, many people spend much time and energy avoiding common, everyday, and unfairly ubiquitous symbols like tunnels and bridges.

Avoidance has a lot of magic in it, which makes it hard to justify—either to other people, who so kindly explain that it's only a little green garter snake and can't possibly hurt you, or to ourselves, who must agree that the damned thing *is* harmless and then have to find some excuse to leave anyway. Since nobody likes having to admit to himself that he's behaving like a fool, avoidance tends to be ignored on a conscious level, at least by the phobic, who may simply refuse to see that he's arranged his whole life around keeping away from his phobia.

It is always possible to some extent to rationalize your avoidance, but this too can get out of hand—as, for instance, when you hear yourself insist you'd rather walk up eight flights than take the elevator because you need the exercise. Remarks like these are dead giveaways. On the other hand, you have plenty of time to get over feeling ashamed of yourself while you're trudging up all those stairs.

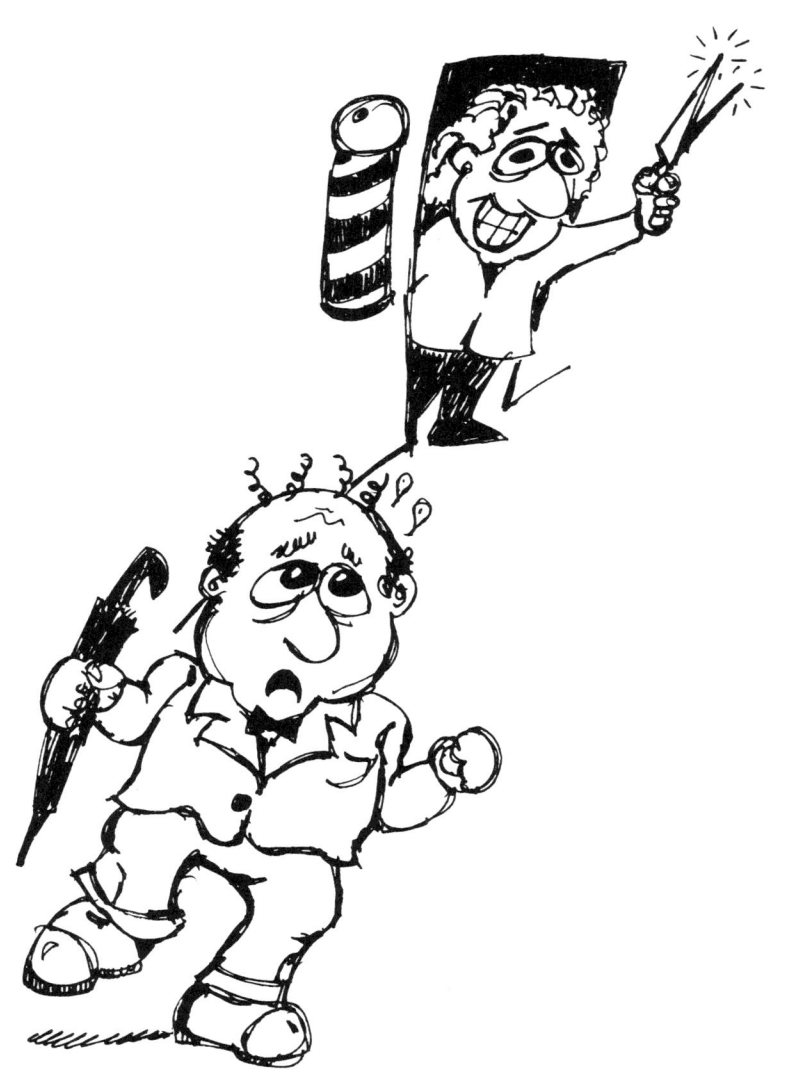

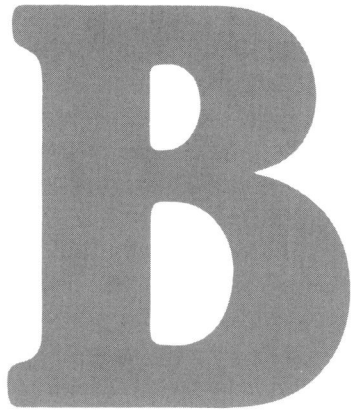

*B is for Behaviorists
Who offer relaxation
To phobics who come looking for
Some desensitization*

BEHAVIORISTS

In contrast to psychoanalysts, behavior therapists, at least as far as phobia is concerned, couldn't care less about the unconscious. They maintain instead that phobias are learned responses—that you're morbidly afraid of some situation, object, or idea because you were once badly frightened by it. The more often you were frightened, the more phobic you are today. This theoretical approach at least has the virtue

B

of simplicity, although it undoubtedly lacks much of the finesse and elegance so intrinsic to Viennese charm.

Anyway, let us say that you are a well-nourished, thirty-seven-year-old male who is phobic to spiders. According to behavior theory, this means that at some earlier date in your life you ran afoul of an aggressive spider in a fear-producing situation. This bad scene "conditioned," as they say, your present-day phobic response. It taught you to associate spiders with fear—spiders became your "phobic stimulus"—and from then on, whenever you've seen a spider, you've automatically reacted by getting very tense and anxious.*

Behavior therapists thus naturally try to cure phobics by changing their responses to the phobic stimulus—a process they carefully do not refer to as "reconditioning" as they think it makes them sound too much like used-car salesmen. If you go to a behavior therapist with your spider phobia, therefore, he won't bother exploring your unconscious conflicts, at least not with any real enthusiasm or sense of purpose. Instead, he'll "desensitize" you by using behavioral techniques.

First, of course, like any other doctor, he'll establish a warm personal relationship and settle the fee. Then he'll relax you completely, through hypnosis or drugs. And then, while you're lying there on his couch feeling ever so comfy and safe he'll present you with a series of spider-stimuli (pictures, verbal suggestions, or live specimens), carefully graded from least to most threatening—a trembly, sweet-faced, little old daddy longlegs to start with, let us say; and to end with, a hairy, mean, poisonous tarantula somewhere between the size of a cup and saucer and a small grapefruit.

---

*This amounts to guilt by association, of course, and is basically unfair to the great majority of spiders who don't actually wish to harm you and are probably only seeking affection when they drop into your curds and whey. But that's the way life is, and the sooner young spiders realize they'll meet a lot of injustice in this world, the better off they'll be.

B

By using this technique, he gradually retrains your responses so that you are conditioned to associate all spiders with relaxation and pleasure rather than with fright. You will easily be able to tell if your desensitization has been successful or not. If it has, the very first time you see a tarantula after your treatment is over, you will instantly close your eyes, count to three, and sink to the ground in a profound hypnotic trance.

BARBERSHOP PHOBIA

One of the oldest recorded phobias, and the only one mentioned in the Bible. Like all phobics, Samson must have had one hell of a time trying to think of some excuse to give Delilah for not wanting to go to the barbershop—and, as so very often happens, when she finally did take one of his stories seriously he was sorry he ever mentioned it.

Psychoanalysts have linked barbershop phobia to a variety of personal problems: fear of scrutiny by others, which is related to agoraphobia; rebelliousness against social customs (there was a time, Virginia, and not too long ago either, when our society made no bones about expecting all its men to get their hair cut at least once every two weeks, and none of this nonsense about stylists, either); fear of mutilation and/or confinement, which has overtones of claustrophobia (*which see*); impatience with delays; anxious experiences with barberlike chairs at the dentist; anxiety over issues of seniority ("It's *my* next!"), and the consequent guilt imposed by a superego that is always eager to tell you you've been a bit too aggressive; and, in those few men who are born queer for the smell of bay rum, a fear of becoming sexually aroused in public for no good or obvious reason. All in all, there seems to be something there for everybody, and it's no wonder that barbers are always complaining about how bad business is.

BIRD PHOBIA

Bird phobia (*see* Symbol; you might also try to catch *Guest in the House* and *The Birds* if they're ever revived on television, since they're both about bird phobia). A morbid dread of our feathered friends; really severe cases won't even eat fried chicken.

Birds are very big as symbolic figures in all cultures, being used to represent every kind of idea you can think of from the Holy Ghost to the United States of America. It's not surprising that birds should be used so often, since—as every bird phobic knows—there isn't any place you can go where there isn't some kind of bird or other like a native haunt.

A bird in flight is universally associated with instinctual freedom and guiltless gratification—what may be called the uninhibited, hail-to-thee-blithe-spirit aspect of birdwatching. This association makes any bird an obvious choice for displacing a personal unconscious conflict onto; since it's culturally acceptable as a symbol of instinctive behavior, why not use it? Consequently, birds are very popular (if that's the right word) phobic objects, and a morbid dread of birds is one of the most common phobias. As a matter of fact, according to one British survey, birds rank right up there at the top along with closed spaces, open spaces, and death as sources of unrealistic fear and terror. So much for your bluebird of happiness.

B

As usual, people who are phobic to birds will stoop to any rationalization to account for their otherwise unaccountable terror. Birds have cruel beaks, they'll tell you; or scratchy sharp claws; or they make a lot of noise, they're dirty, their feathers fall off. One woman, hard pressed by a feeder-filling nature lover to explain her dislike, said defiantly, "I hate birds because they eat beneficial insects."

Like every phobic object, birds must carry projected guilt as well as displaced temptation—guilt that makes them seem both anxiety-provoking and undesirable. In this area birds are especially difficult to deal with. They're not like tunnels and bridges and tall buildings, all of which can generally be counted on to remain in one place, so that you can more or less easily avoid them if you happen to be phobic to them. Birds are different, mainly because they're alive. They have minds of their own, however small, and they are always in motion, flying this way and that. *Free as a bird* also means unpredictable, uncontrollable, and consequently—very often—unavoidable as a bird. "Don't try to tell me they're harmless," one phobic said testily. "If they're not out to get me, why are they always aiming themselves to fly directly at my head?"

BLUSHING

Blushing. See Erythrophobia.

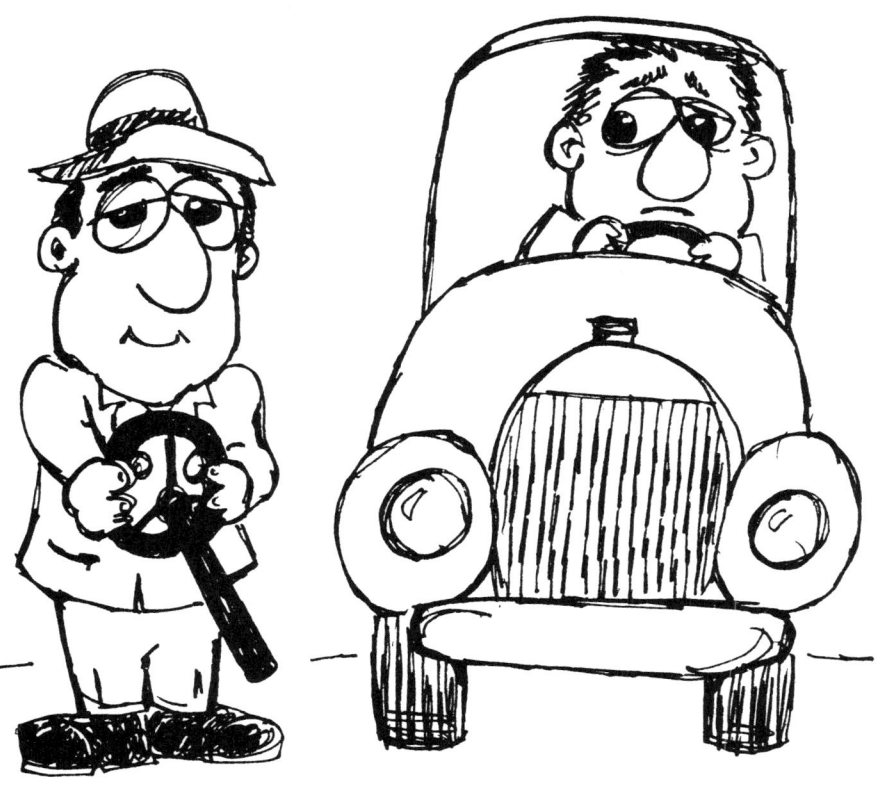

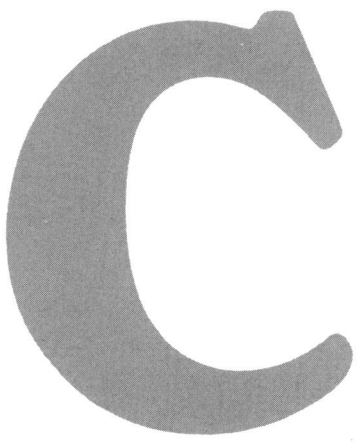

> *When you bravely embrace*
> *The thing you most dread*
> *It seems Counterphobia's*
> *Turning your head*

COUNTERPHOBIA

Some phobics, after having displaced their instinctual conflict onto a symbolic object, situation, or idea, defend themselves against their projected anxiety not by avoidance *(which see)* but by counterphobic behavior: that is, they continually—although unconsciously, which differentiates what they do from action therapy—seek out and confront what they're phobic to as a way of making believe they

C

aren't afraid at all. A child who is unable to admit to himself that he has a morbid dread of fire plays with matches. An adult who can't admit to himself that he's acrophobic takes up skydiving.

Thus, although on the surface counterphobia is the opposite of avoidance, it actually serves exactly the same underneath and magical purpose—mastering the guilty fear attached to an unconscious temptation. Which of these two defensive ploys is chosen seems to be a matter of personality. The people who find counterphobia attractive are generally those who are ashamed to admit weakness—Leos, say, who are willing to die a lot (if necessary, a little bit at a time) just to prove to the world they really are the masters of their fates and the captains of their souls. Sometimes this dying is more than a figure of speech, for the same desperate need to deny fear that drives men to counterphobia is also one of the reasons they do foolishly heroic things like throw themselves on live hand grenades.

Counterphobics tend to brag about their courage, which is especially understandable since nobody else thinks they're brave because nobody else knows the real situation. Take Don Juan, for instance: a classic example of counterphobic behavior. The poor man was probably suffering from a severe parthenophobia—a morbid fear of virgins—but, as we all know, instead of avoiding these symbolic objects he sought them out with the compulsive, irrational insistence typical of counterphobia, then went around boasting about his conquests afterward to anyone who would listen. The fact is, though, he bragged mostly to remind himself how much of a hero he was. And his lists of the women he'd seduced amounted to awarding himself citations for bravery for having occupied all those square yards of enemy territory.

Unfortunately, counterphobia, like all magic, cannot be depended on. It simply doesn't last. The phobic has to keep

C

repeating his counterphobic actions because he can never convince himself he's not anxious or afraid, which is not surprising because he really *is* anxious and afraid. At best, therefore, counterphobic behavior amounts (and especially for a Don Juan) to a stopgap measure.

Furthermore, the real-world situation may change so that the counterphobia has to be abandoned—and then where are you? If you're an acrophobic skydiver and get permanently grounded, or if you're a Don Juan and the supply of virgins runs out (a situation that today seems all too likely a prospect and in the near future, too), it means that you have to think up a whole new counterphobic pattern. Which is a bit of a bore—especially since the chances are you're at an age when you're no longer as inventive or flexible as you used to be.

CHILDHOOD PHOBIAS

Childhood phobias (*see* Little Hans). The morbid dreads of childhood—not to be confused with the morbid dread of children, the proper name for which is pedophobia (*see* Nomenclature)—are usually transitory, but while they last they're as intense and painful as any adult phobia. Children can be and are phobic to practically anything—animals, the dark, vacuum cleaners, fire sirens, injections, doctors, loud noises, policemen, feathers, toilets, sleep, ghosts and other mysteries, strangers, space, and heights. Many childhood phobias go relatively unnoticed, because parents know that every kid has "normal" fears, and they also know that he's supposed to outgrow his anxieties. If not, he'll suppress them,

—hopefully so that they don't reappear till much later when he's all grown up and his phobias are no longer his parents' responsibility.

One situational phobia of childhood has, however, received a great deal of professional attention: school phobia. A child who is unendurably anxious about going to school usually has a lot of ambivalence about being separated from his mother: he both wants and doesn't want to grow up. The mother of such a child is also ambivalent about seeing her baby leave her, and her anxieties reinforce his. This is probably the only known phobia where two people have to understand what's going on before anybody grows out of anything, and most experts recommend that both mother and child go into treatment. Although not necessarily together.

CLAUSTROPHOBIA

A morbid dread of enclosed spaces—tunnels, closets, airplanes, windowless offices, subways, boats, elevators, trains, automobiles, coffins, tight clothes. As even this partial list indicates, there are two main varieties of claustrophobia: in one of them you're afraid of being trapped inside a non-moving space, like a closet; in the other, of being trapped inside a space that's moving, like a subway car.

In either of these situations, the anxiety is focused not so much on the enclosure itself as on the idea that you have no way out, that you can't escape or leave whenever you want. At its worst, this sense of being trapped is felt to be the equivalent of suffocation, so that you tend to hold your breath as long as possible just in case there really is no more air available; if necessary you faint so people will move back

C

and let you have whatever extra oxygen may be around. Modern technology makes it possible for today's claustrophobes to know which kind of claustrophobic situation scares them more. It may be of some comfort to find out, for instance, that you're extremely fearful about flying but only mildly worried about being trapped in the toilet once you're aboard the plane. On the other hand, it may not.

Claustrophobia is thought to be related to a couple of different instinctual conflicts. One involves dreading and at the same time desiring to be back inside the mother's body, which may explain (at least to an analyst's satisfaction) why claustrophobia is so frequently associated with fears of suffocation and of the dark.

Another instinctual conflict that theoretically underlies the moving-vehicle brand of claustrophobia has to do with the need to control or escape a mounting excitement (basically sexual) that you also enjoy. You project the anxieties that this situation arouses onto whatever vehicle is stimulating the excitement (which presumably once upon a time must have been your baby carriage), and you fear being trapped in it because that makes you a helpless prisoner of your own excitement which is no longer under your own control. People with this conflict do not willingly go on roller coasters if they go at all, and they also tend to be rather grumpy about being held down and tickled.

The claustrophobic dread of being trapped is the main source of terror for those who are phobic about flying, and not, as you might think, any fear of heights. Because he needs to feel he's in control, the only truly ideal way for a severely claustrophobic person to travel (besides walking) is to drive himself, preferably not too fast, so he knows he can stop the car whenever he wants to. Subways, buses, and trains may be manageable if he doesn't get too anxious to believe that the next station does exist, or to remember that if (or rather

C

when) worst does come to worst, he can always pull the emergency cord and get off to breathe again.

Once you're on a plane, though, and they've raised that drawbridge and slammed the portcullis behind you, you've had it—the whole thing is completely out of your hands and you're up and away with no possibility of getting out until somebody else you don't even see says you can. Providing that he's able to find the airport before you run out of fuel, or that the wings don't fall off en route, or that the engines, one of which is definitely making a funny noise, don't catch on fire first. Or all three.

Have a drink. Since things are already as bad as they can get, have two. Have a tranquilizer. They're small—have two. Try listening to the stereo. Many claustrophobes find that soothing music distracts them enough to make a difference, and plug in their earphones as soon as they sit down. If you're one of these, just be sure you check the program guide first, because some man who didn't reports that he tuned in while the plane was taxiing out to the runway and a large symphony orchestra immediately began playing *Taps* into both sides of his head. He fainted, of course. And though he doesn't recommend it as a way to go, at least for once in his life he was able to say he'd really relaxed on a plane.

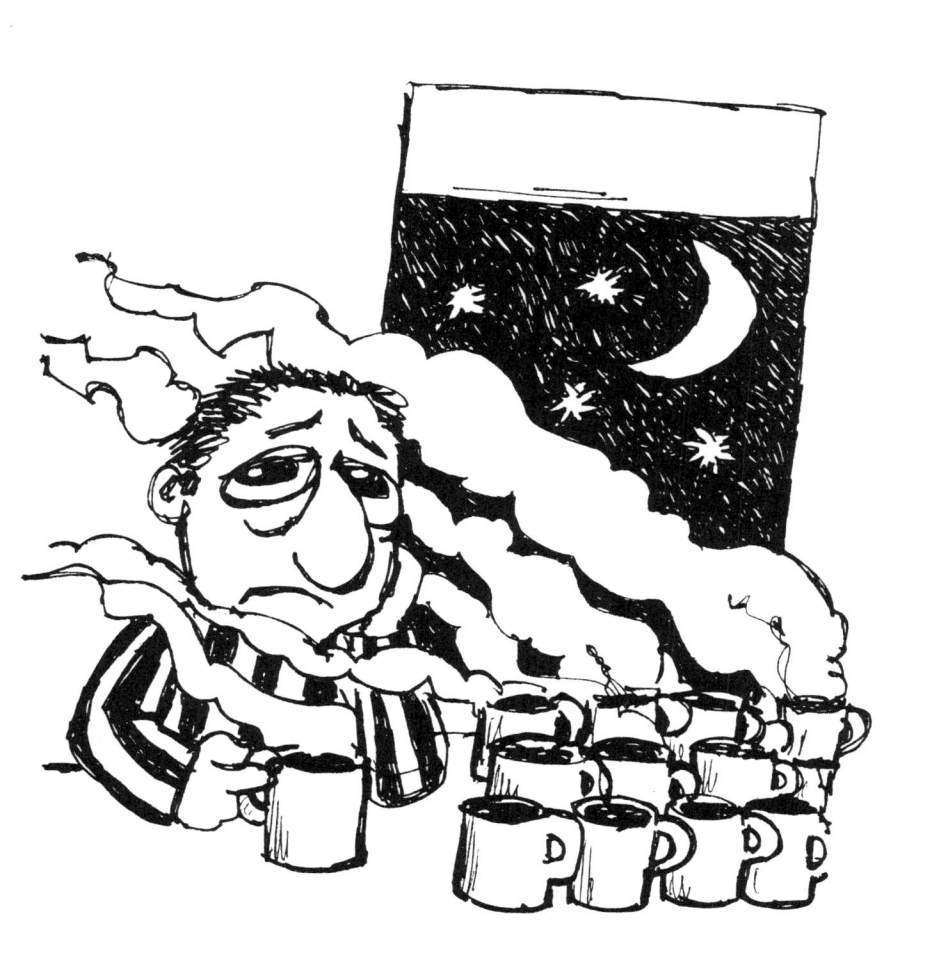

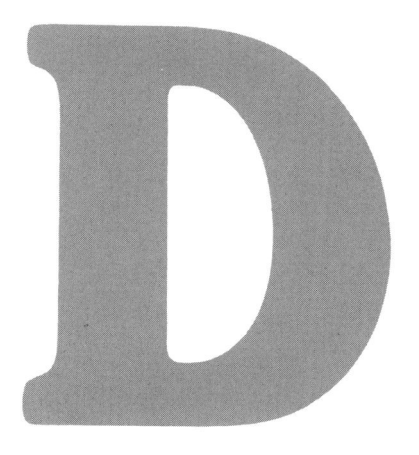

D is for Displacement,
A symbolic substitution
Made when inner conflict
Can have no resolution.

An idea or an object
That your mind accepts as equal
Becomes your own anxiety
And phobia's the sequel.

DISPLACEMENT

The transfer of psychic energy, including emotional energy, from a threatening or unpleasant unconscious idea to a substitute idea more acceptable to your conscious mind. In phobia the unconscious idea is theoretically an instinctual

D

conflict heavily laden with guilt and anxiety, which God knows is not anything you'd want to dwell on. But it doesn't go away by itself, either—which leaves it up to your conscious mind to find some place to dump it.

Which is just about what happens: you select some thing that for your own entirely and usually unconscious personal reasons you can consider an equivalent idea, object, or situation, and displace onto it the emotional energy that rightfully belongs to your unconscious conflict. By so doing you have created a phobic object for yourself. Congratulations.

Unfortunately, displacement solves only half your problem. Although you've now fixed it so that the idea that so offends your conscious mind remains hidden, your original anxiety has become both visible and concrete, embodied in the phobic object. That's why you panic so unreasonably, even though you know that it isn't going to hurt you: your unconscious is reacting to the terror that it knows lies behind or underneath this symbol, and there's nothing your conscious mind can do to make you feel better except to direct you to get the hell out of there as soon as possible.

DEATH PHOBIA

A morbid dread of death—and hell to live with. People who have a death phobia are continually and consciously afraid that they'll die at any minute, which as you can well imagine tends to put a damper on cheerful conversation. Any activity may be threatening—you can be poisoned by what you eat, sexual intercourse is physically strenuous, your friends are going to infect you with their diseases, and even your own heart can turn on you.

D

Death-phobic people are not the same as hypochondriacs, because they're not worried about being ill or even keeping themselves healthy; they're worried about dying. Nor are they suicidal—just the opposite. The idea of death fills them with terror, and they're not in the least tempted to get it over with. The point is that the concept of death serves exactly the same symbolic function as any other phobic object or situation: it represents on the level of consciousness another and less acceptable idea. In some cases, apparently, the idea of death stands for loss of love or loneliness; in others it seems to represent a punishment for having wished other people dead, for which the phobics' consciences penalize them by making them turn this aggression against themselves. How's that for getting even?

DIRT PHOBIA

Dirt phobia. See Misophobia.

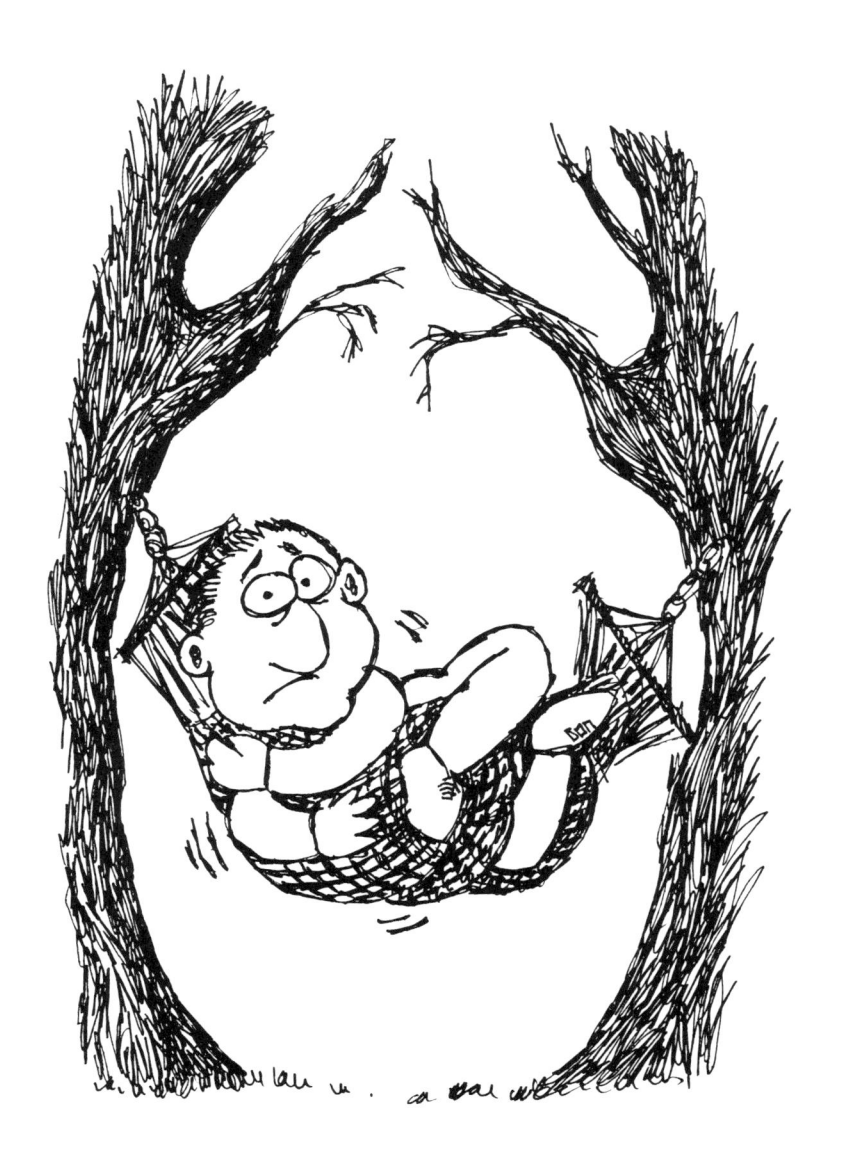

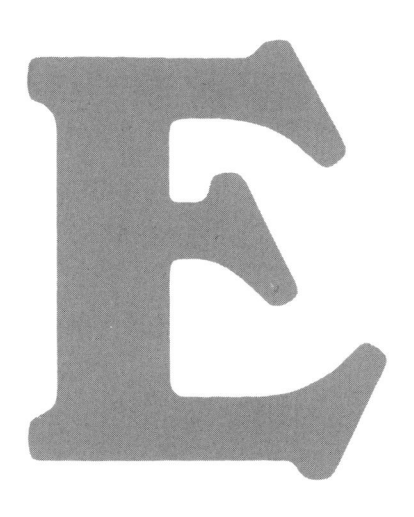

EQUILIBRIUM PHOBIAS

Morbid dread of situations that affect the sense of equilibrium: amusement-park rides, roller coasters, swings, teeter-totters, light shows, excessive speeds, small boats in rough waters, and vibrating chairs.

Equilibrium phobia is experienced as the usual kind of mental anguish, of course, but it may also suffer a sea change into a physical symptom: seasickness, nausea, vertigo, dizziness. Very often you get both at once, which doesn't seem fair.

The underlying conflict, like that in some varieties of claustrophobia *(which see)* is thought to be a struggle against and a desire for an unacceptably high degree of (sexual)

E

excitement. You're really afraid of the threat posed by losing control of your own dangerously thrilling impulses. You tiger, you.

Like all phobias, equilibrium phobias are noticeably irrational and have nothing to do with realistic danger. This kind of phobic would rather walk among a school of sharks in shallow water than have to swing in a hammock slung between two trees over a mattress on dry land.

ERYTHROPHOBIA

A morbid dread of blushing. This condition isn't as rare as you might think, but doesn't ordinarily occur by itself. Instead, it's usually part of severe stage fright or one of the symptoms associated with agoraphobia.

Someone who is terrified of blushing is essentially struggling with an intense desire to be exhibitionistically aggressive. He wants to demand that everyone notice, applaud, and admire him, but at the same time he fears being punished for wishing to be so powerful.

It's pretty clear, of course, that erythrophobes are very conceited. They are so sure they're among the world's most beautiful and charming people that they believe the mere sight of their faces will strike an audience dead in its tracks. Like Medusa, they believe their very looks can kill. And they blush to admit it.

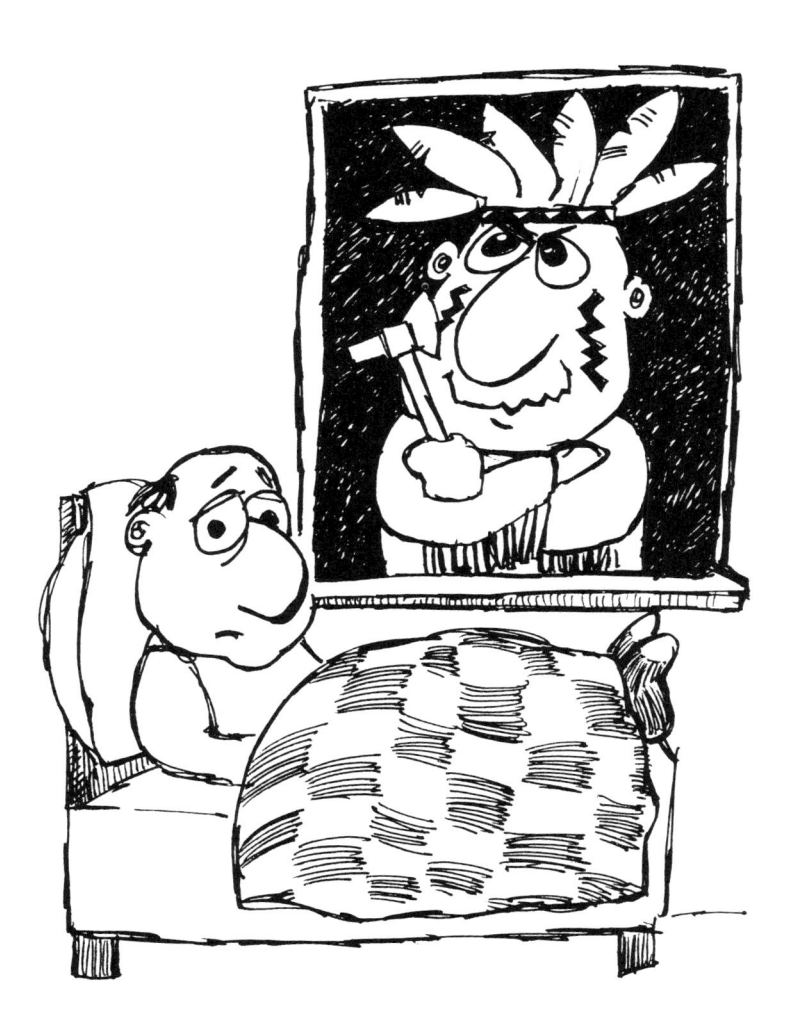

F

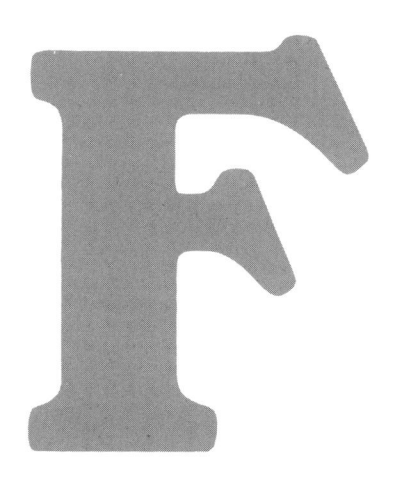

Fear-trees growing
Evergreen
Are seldom few
And phobia-tween

In case you're not already anxious enough, this is perhaps as good a place as any to mention that if phobic fears are left unwatched, they tend to flourish and spread like the green bay tree or creeping sedum. Because a phobia is essentially a defense, not a solution, it doesn't get rid of the basic conflict —it only allows you to sidestep it. Furthermore, a phobia may be so ridiculous that you're ashamed to admit, even to yourself, that feathers send you into a panic. Which means you ignore the existence of your anxiety as much as possible without even realizing it.

In general, though, an unsolved conflict and an overlooked

F

anxiety are going to get worse rather than better. First it's feathers, which isn't so terrible. Next thing you know you find that Indian headdresses make you uneasy. Then you start worrying about seeing a molting bird. Then it's a dead pheasant in a butcher's window, then a down pillow with a hole in it, then an overstuffed sofa, and you end up sitting on a plain wooden bench and sleeping under a rag rug. A little fear may go a far way.

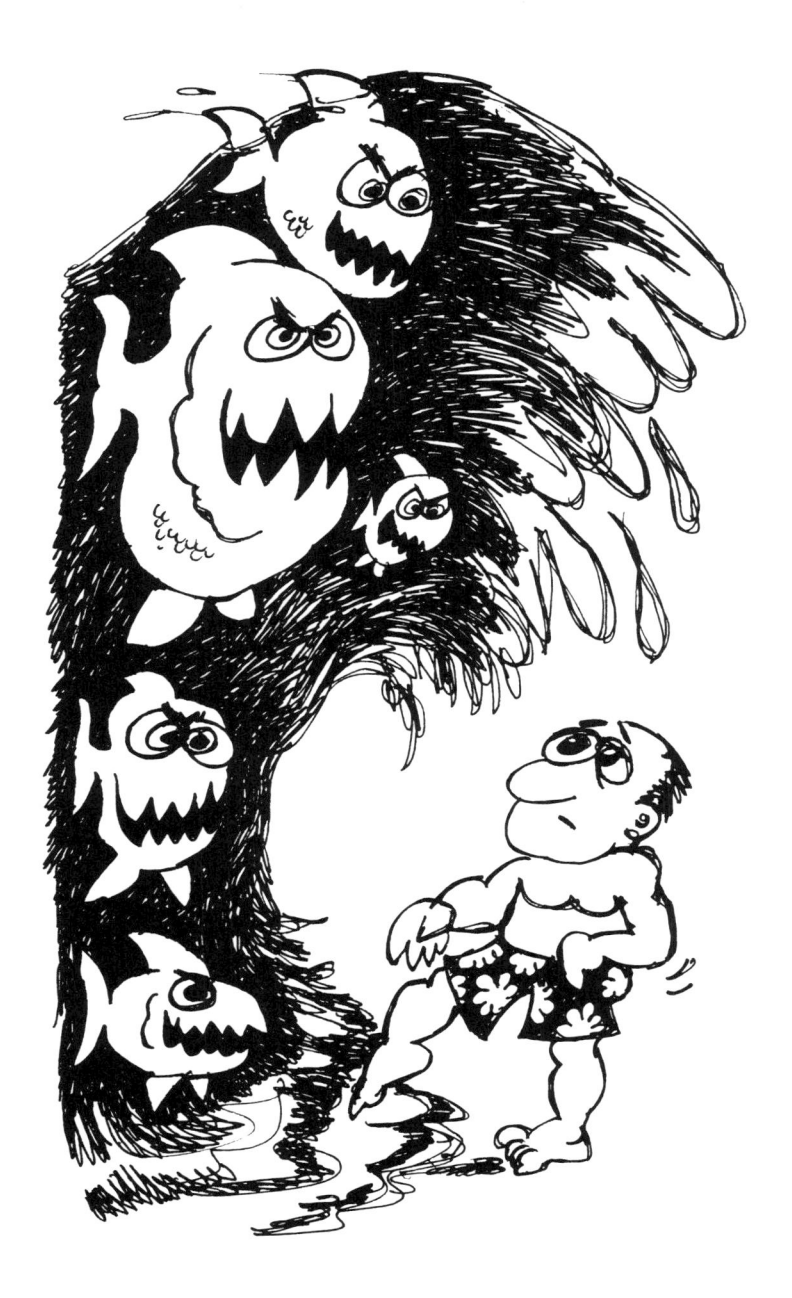

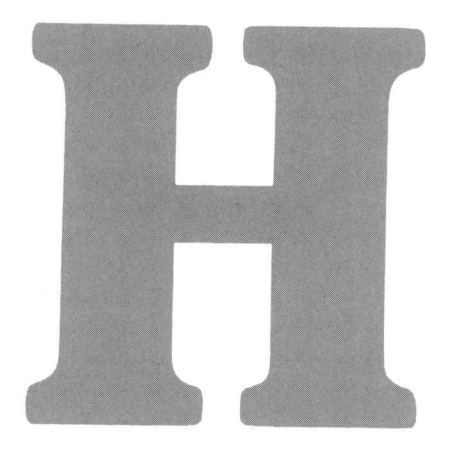

HEIGHTS

Heights. See Acrophobia.

HYDROPHOBIA

A morbid dread of water—anything from the sight of water dripping from a faucet to an entire ocean. Children may incur hydrophobia if they've been scared by surf or been ducked too much and held under too deep, and the aversion may stay

H

with them for life, since it's practically never really necessary to go in swimming even if you're at the beach in a suit.

Hydrophobia is also one of the symptoms of rabies, which is a virus disease affecting the brain. This kind of hydrophobia is easily differentiated from the purely mental kind, because you get it from being bitten by a rabid animal—dog, wolf, chipmunk, squirrel, cat—which is surely something you would notice and remember. Furthermore, the other clinical symptoms of rabies include melancholy, irritation, sexual indulgence and assault, alcoholism, violent rage, and convulsions, all of which are hard to overlook.

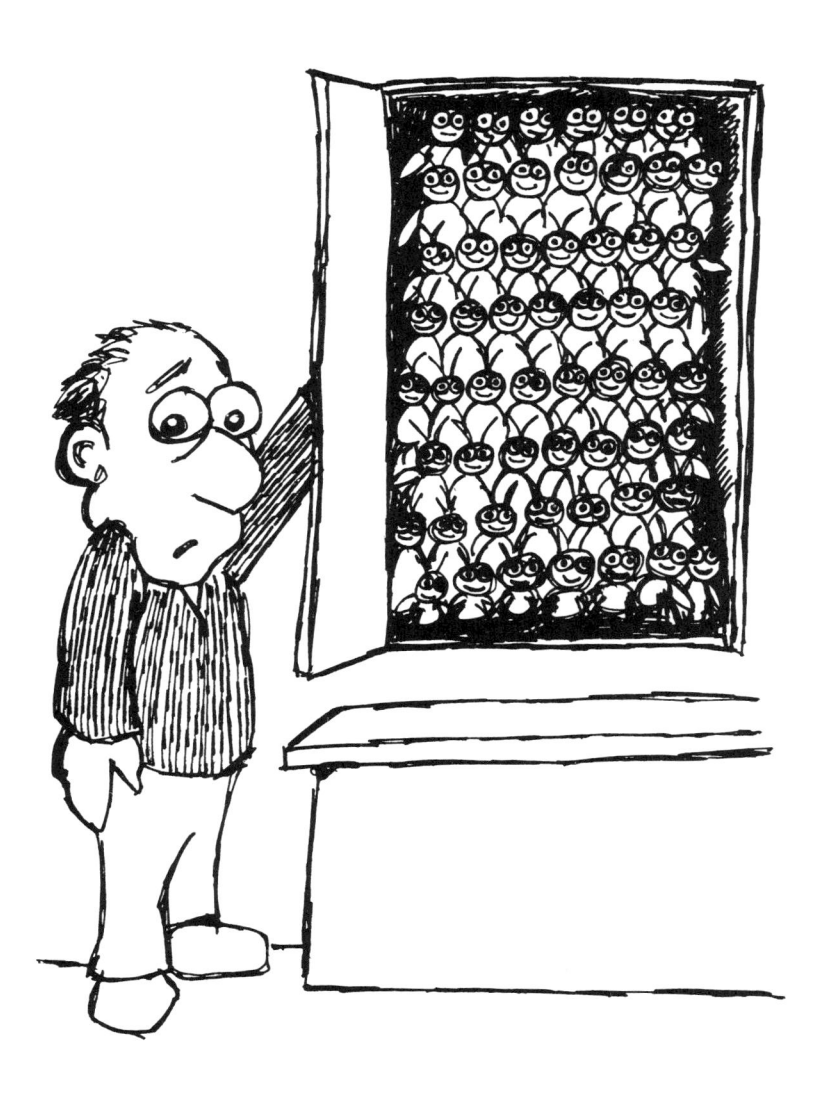

I

Now doth the busy little bee
Succumb to bombs of DDT
Nor ants nor roaches get away
From phobics who do kneel to spray

INSECT PHOBIA

A morbid dread of insects—creepy, crawly, buzzy, squirmy, stingy, zooming, itchy, biting, unpredictable, ubiquitous, ugly, big or little bugs. Insect phobias come in almost as many varieties as insects do. Some people are phobic to moths but not butterflies, others to insects that crawl but not to fliers, some to big bugs but not to small; others loathe the

I

soft-bodied, squashy kind but claim that the crunchy ones like beetles and ants don't bother them. Much.

Many insects have achieved symbolic status in our culture. Bees are continually being held up as examples of the thrifty virtues and the dangerous tempers inherent in an anal-sadistic nature. Moths and butterflies connote the feminine qualities of frivolous, fickle beauty; we scare ourselves with songs about Poor Butterfly and fables of moths being destroyed by flames, reminding ourselves thereby that like them we too are here today and gone tomorrow. And spiders have a bad reputation for being unloving mothers and castrating wives. A spider not only doesn't take care of her children, she also devours her spouse and then proceeds to live happily alone, spinning her webs and waiting for the next generation of victims.

Which doesn't necessarily mean that you're phobic to spiders because you're unconsciously afraid of being eaten alive by your mother as a punishment for wanting to make love to her. Of course not. On the other hand, you might ask yourself what has she done to you lately?

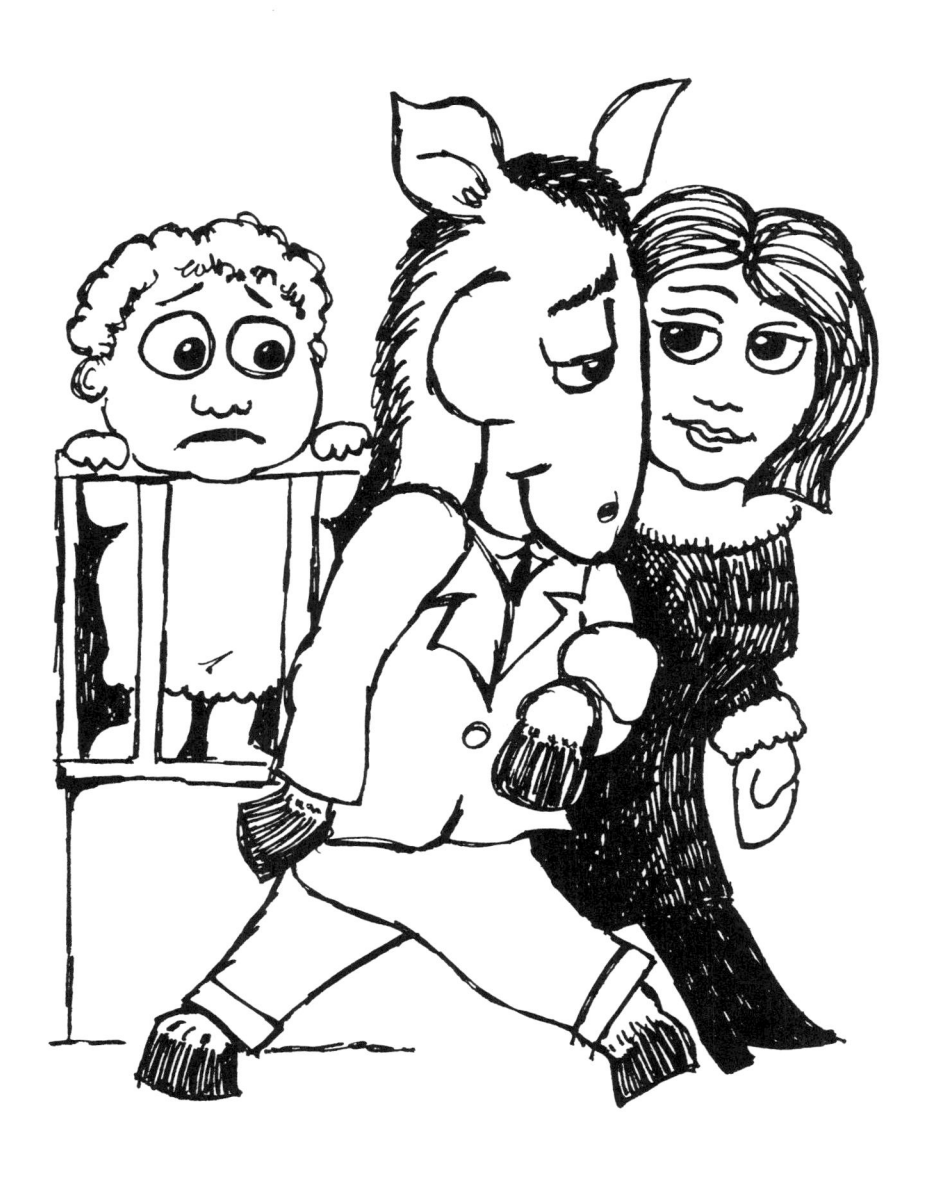

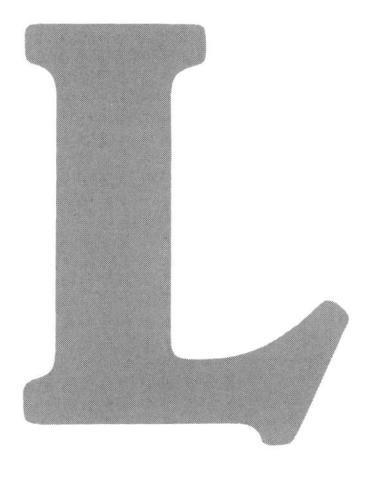

Sometimes a boy's best friend is his horse.
—*Sigmund Freud*

LITTLE HANS

Little Hans was a Viennese who achieved lasting fame very early in life when his case history was published in 1909 by Sigmund Freud as "Analysis of a Phobia in a Five Year Old Boy."* Hans grew up to become a fairly well-known stage designer, but as far as analysts are concerned, nothing he did

---

*Little Hans of Vienna was not, you may be sure, his real name. Freud was always very careful to protect his patients from unwanted notoriety, and hence when he published his papers scrupulously falsified everybody's identity except, of course, his own.

later on is half as important as the fact that between the ages of three and five he was phobic to horses.

Briefly, as Freud first got the story from the kid's dad, little Hans was in terrible trouble and his parents were at their wits' end. (Don't forget, advances in modern transportation have today made hippophobia more or less easy to live with, but in 1909 Vienna, like every other metropolis, was Horse City.) Hans had decided that he couldn't stand the sight of a horse; in a sense this was his basic mistake, for he could no more avoid seeing or meeting a horse whenever he went outside than he could sprout wings and fly. Consequently he had taken to spending most of his time indoors, teasing his baby sister, pestering the maid, and getting on his mother's nerves to the point where she felt something drastic had to be done. She'd gotten so upset, as a matter of fact, that she'd sent her husband to see a psychiatrist—and that's how Freud happened to get involved in the case to begin with.

The big difficulty, actually, as it always does with phobias, lay in the fact that Hans' family simply did not understand that his panic was real. Since his mother and father weren't the least bit afraid of horses themselves, and none of their friends was afraid of horses, and none of their friends' *children* was afraid of horses, they didn't see any reason for Hans to be afraid. This argument made very little impression on Hans and did nothing to change his behavior—but his parents still thought it was relevant and used it on every possible occasion.

When they finally saw that Hans was not going to stop being afraid of horses because nobody else was afraid, they told themselves that he would grow out of it in a couple of weeks. When *that* didn't happen, they decided it was time to take the matter seriously. Hans was going to have to confront and conquer his fears—or they, as good Austrian parents, would know the reason why. They determined to teach him

L

just how silly he was, and after some thought they hit upon a properly Germanic pedagogical method, combining kindly ridicule, complete lack of sympathy, and rigorous logic. It's not that they didn't love him, you understand—but they were action therapists at heart, and totally dedicated to making him conform for his own good.

It is simple enough to imagine a typical episode in this phase of Hans' phobia. The scene is played in the street outside Hans' house. He and his mother appear in the doorway. Gripping his reluctant hand firmly in her own, she hauls him down the immaculate front stoop, across the newly washed sidewalk, and over the cobblestones to the opposite side of the road where some feckless delivery boy has parked an enormous Percheron dray horse, easily twenty hands high at the shoulder. She lifts him up so he'll be as close to the monster as possible.

"Say hello to the horsie, Hans. *Nice* horsie."

Hans trembles and shuts his eyes as tight as he can.

"Doesn't little Hans want to kiss the lovely great big horsie on his beautiful soft black velvet nose?"

Hans shakes his head emphatically.

"Just once for Mamma?"

Not a chance.

"How do you know you don't like it if you won't even try?"

Hans does his best to crawl into the space between her shoulder and neck, and begins to whimper.

"There's nothing to cry about, you big baby! Watch. See, Mamma is going to kiss the nice gentle horsie right smack on his big black velvet nosie so he'll make friends with silly little Hans. *Mamma* isn't afraid."

Hans emits piercing shrieks at irregular intervals until eventually even a Teutonic mother has to give up, take him home, and put him to bed with a cold cloth on his forehead. During all this disagreeable and undignified squabbling about

L

whether or not his big black velvet nosie is going to be kissed or not, and if so by whom, the horse—who underneath his massive *sangfroid* happens to be extremely sensitive to rejection—has been carelessly tossing his mane and pretending to be very much interested in whether or not all his shoes are on tight. The sight of little Hans being carried off kicking and screaming breaks his spirit, however; and when the delivery boy reappears and tells him to gee-up, he hangs his head and wearily trudges on, barely able to drag his wagon back to the stable where he remains off his feed for the next couple of days, struggling to work through painful feelings of depression, guilt, anomie, and loss of self-esteem.

As any phobic could predict, a few more of these sturdy no-nonsense attempts to teach him that horses were his friends, and little Hans began refusing to get out of bed in the morning at all, let alone go outside the house. Furthermore, his phobia showed ominous signs of spreading to include giraffes and elephants. This development proved to be the last straw as far as Hans' father was concerned. He gave up logic in favor of psychology, and agreed to his wife's urging to go consult Freud.

It only took a few sessions with Freud before the father felt free enough to ask Hans what it was about horses that scared him so much—a question that neither parent had ever bothered to ask. After the usual amount of hemming and hawing, Hans finally confessed that the reason horses scared him was that they were so big and had black muzzles and wore shades in front of their eyes, and besides they stumbled and fell down in the street. Hans' father duly relayed this information to Freud, and everything immediately became crystal-clear, for Freud had already observed that Hans' father wore eyeglasses and had a big black mustache.*

Hans' associations (huge size, that is, huge to him: blinders—glasses; black nose—mustache) were certainly transparent enough for Freud to conclude that Hans was not actually afraid of horses at all (surprise!), but that instead he was—for the usual Oedipal reasons, of course—unconsciously afraid of his father and had displaced his angry, hateful feelings, plus the guilty fears these feelings evoked, *plus* his fears of being punished for wanting his mother, onto horses. This left him free to like his father, but as we have seen sure raised hell with his playtime outdoors.

Under Freud's guidance the father was able to dispel his son's terror until eventually Hans came to feel only a mild dislike for horses, which everyone agreed was a big improvement. Chances are, though, that Hans never got to the point of kissing one on his big black velvet nosie—for the chances also are that even after he grew up, he still harbored some Oedipal resentments, and never forgave his father for being there first. Nobody does.

---

*Freud does not tell us whether or not the father also stumbled and fell down in the street. However, we may rest assured that he certainly would have included this significant detail in his paper if the father—who, all things considered, quite possibly may have been doing a bit of drinking now and then—had seen fit to mention it.

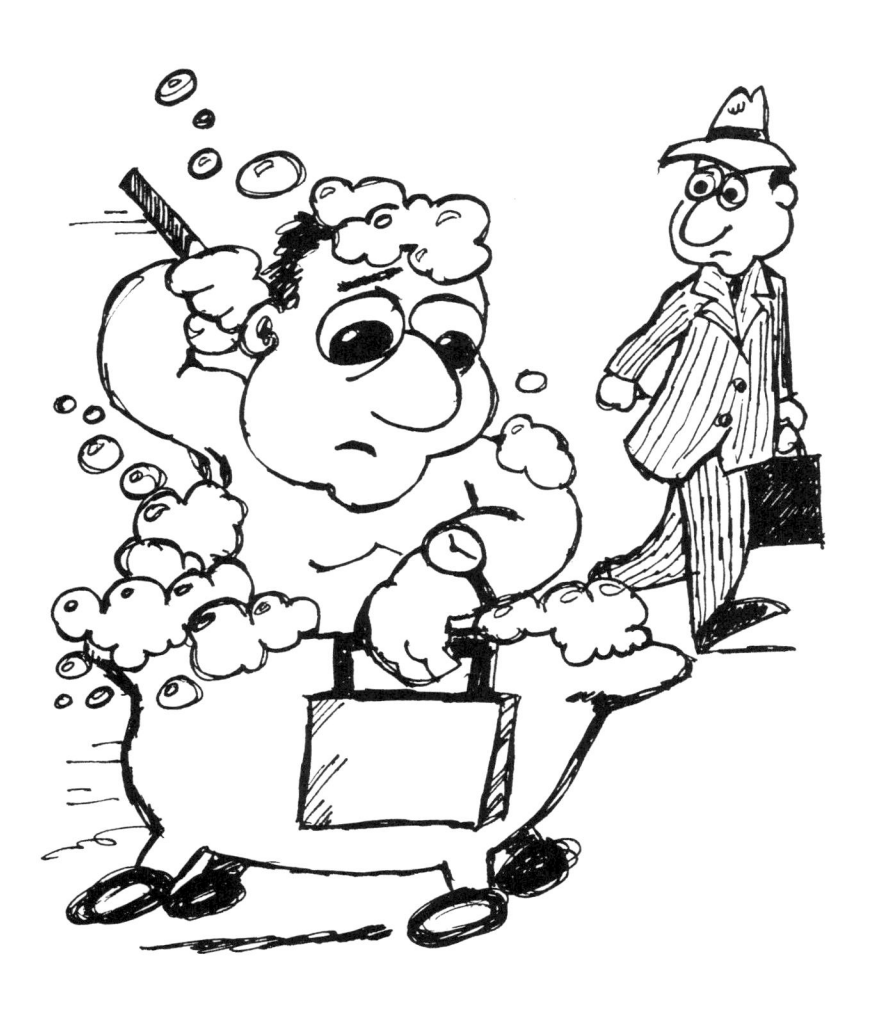

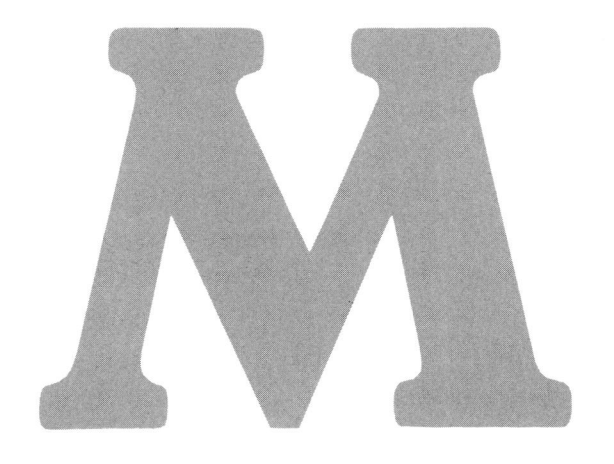

MISOPHOBIA

A morbid dread of contamination of any kind—dirt, dust, germs, radiation, disease, infection, plague, and pestilence. Mildly misophobic people are splendidly clean housekeepers. Their telephones get disinfected after every call, their floors are scrubbed till they shine, their furniture is *always* dusted, and they will not let you help with the dishes because you're not fussy enough for them. A severely misophobic person cannot go out in public without a gauze surgical mask, and is usually not terribly popular because he won't shake hands, which makes everybody else feel like Typhoid Mary. Which, to a misophobe, they are.

M

This is one phobia that has to be watched very carefully, because, what with pollution and all, it's bound to get worse. Furthermore, misophobes are continually being reminded that there is yet more to do, since Madison Avenue is always finding some new way to scare consumers into feeling dirty so they'll buy more deodorants and soap. Which is really very hard on a misophobe, who as it is spends all day up to the elbows in detergents and anxiety. The last thing she needs is to be told that she only *thinks* she's immaculate.

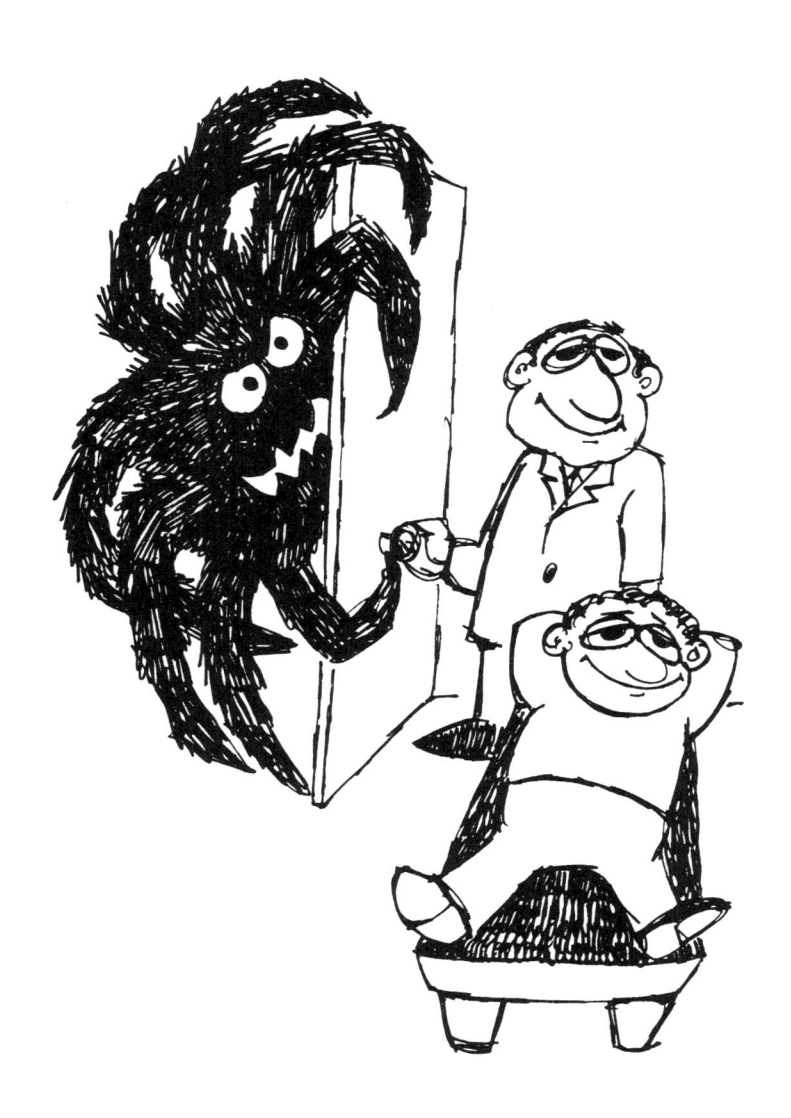

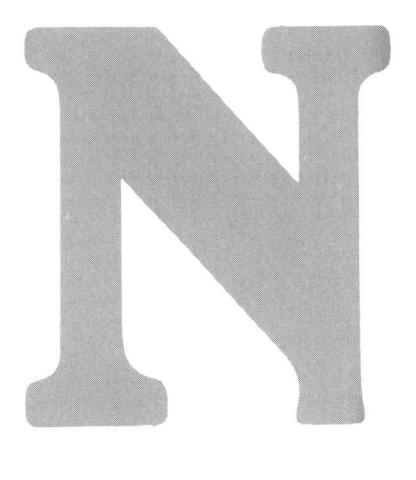

NOMENCLATURE

Even the casual reader has probably noticed by now that *phobia* and *phobic* crop up on almost every page of this book, and has more than likely asked himself the significance of these two words. It's not difficult to define them. *Phobia* means "fear." And although a *phobic* is not really a coward or even a poltroon—not one of your regular run-of-the-Milquetoasts at all—he is most definitely someone who's afraid (*see* Anxiety).

Both *phobia* and *phobic*, like so many other medical terms, come from the Greek. Modern medicine certainly does owe an enormous debt of gratitude to those ancient Greek physicians who could have spent their nights treating sick patients

N

but instead were willing to sit around in cafés for long hours on hard stone benches, drinking *ouzo* and making up names for diseases. Long before anybody else had begun to worry about what to call things, these devoted and zealous doctors had done it all for us—and for all time, too.

As a result of their activity, in order to name a phobia, what you have to do is first look up the Greek word for the phobic object in your handy little pocket Greek dictionary of medical terminology, then tack phobia on the end of it. That way, a morbid fear of bees becomes melissophobia; of tuna fish, thynnophobia; of flycatchers, phoebeophobia, and so on. It's as easy as rolling off a log once you catch on to how to do it, and besides, the medical profession being as conservative as it is, it's roughly twenty-two hundred years too late to think about doing anything else.

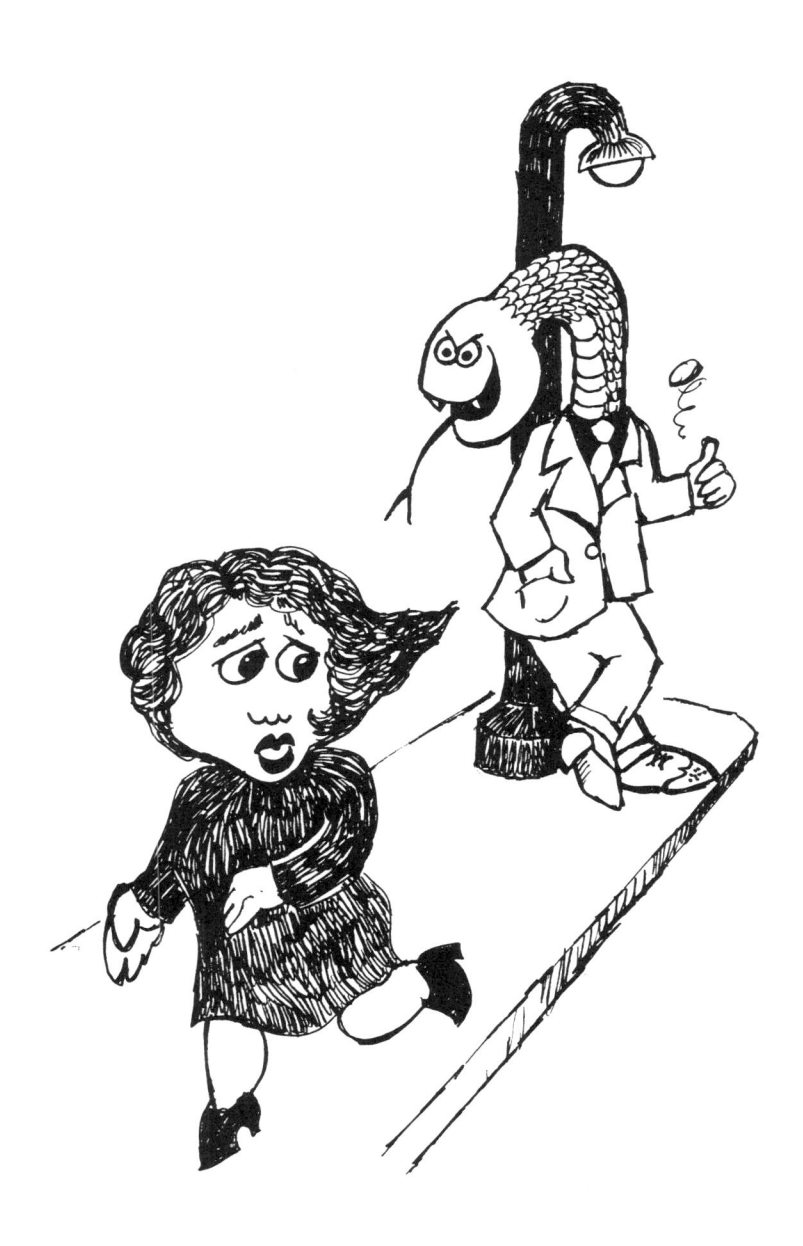

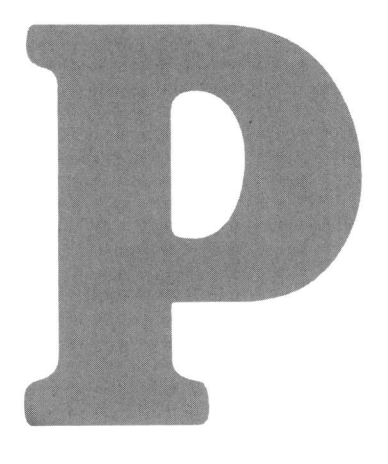

*What is phobia? Who is she
That all our brains pretend her?*

PHOBIA

This condition can be defined in one simple little word—*fear* (*see also* Anxiety *and* Nomenclature)—which certainly does seem clear enough. However, when it comes to describing what *kind* of fear, it gets to be a little like trying to locate a mythical Balkan kingdom on the map of Asia. As a psychological symptom, phobia is one of those gray areas whose boundaries are so vague that it's hardly ever in the same place two days in a row.

On the one hand, you see, phobia merges imperceptibly

into the fears attached to obsession and compulsion, with both of which it has much in common. On the other hand, it's not easily distinguished from morbid delusion and paranoia, in addition to which it also shows regrettable similarities to some aspects of anxiety hysteria and superstition. However, it's in there somewhere—we do know that all right. Perhaps drifting lazily a little to the north of the Isles of Langerhans. Or perhaps not.

So much for psychophysiological geography. Let us now consider what causes this interesting mental condition. The truth is, nobody really *knows* what causes it, or why some of us are phobic and others are not. Several alternative psychological theories have been proposed, however, and in the interests of advancing scientific knowledge you are asked to choose between them here. In Question A please check the explanation you think is closest to the truth, and state briefly the reasons for your choice. In Question B you are given the opportunity to explain yourself at length in an essay-type answer. All ready? Please see the facing page.

P

QUESTION A:
I believe I am phobic because of (check one)
- [ ] 1. Bad emotional conditioning. (When I was ―― years old I was frightened by a ―――― when I ――――――. And ever since then I ――――――.)
- [ ] 2. An unconscious (sexual or aggressive) instinctual conflict. (Remember, briefness counts. The computer is programmed for 25 words or less. This questionnaire is not supposed to be a substitute for an analytic session.)
- [ ] 3. A predominance of black bile in my circulatory system.
- [ ] 4. A weak character. (This is merely a descriptive term. No moral, sexual, or toilet-training judgment is implied.)
- [ ] 5. An inherited phlogiston deficiency in my Purkinje cells (the so-called Felmly–Flumster Syndrome).
- [ ] 6. All of these.
- [ ] 7. None of these.

QUESTION B (Extended essay; 25 words or less):
What is your phobia? How do you feel about it? How has it helped you to get ahead? Is there any other symptom you would prefer?

A factor analysis (p greater than .01) reveals that there is one characteristic exhibited by all true phobics: they know that their fear is not rational and experience it as something alien to their basic selves. "I don't have the phobia, exactly—it's more like the phobia has me," as one commendably terse man summed it all up.

We may conclude, therefore, that if you think your irrational fear is even a little bit foolish, you're phobic. But if

P

you think your irrational fear is absolutely justified—if nothing can convince you that shirt buttons do not constitute a genuine threat to your continued existence—then you are not phobic within the true meaning of the term. You're crazy.

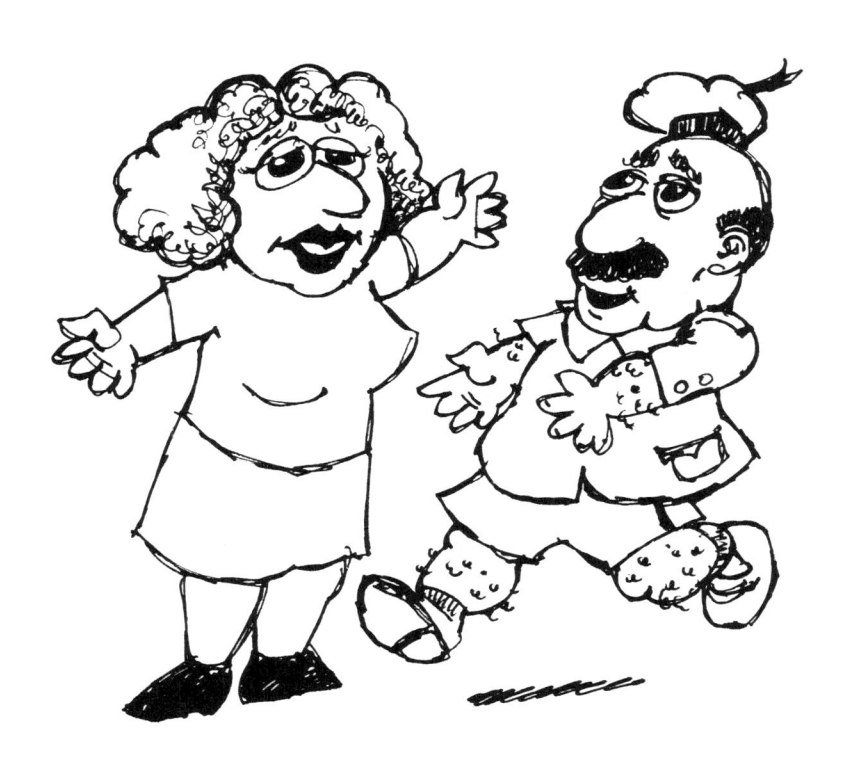

The Lord helps those who help themselves.

RESCUE FANTASIES

Because phobias are magic in action, we have to deal with them by magic. In addition to avoidance and counterphobia, those two major magical insurance policies, most of us find that rescue fantasies—minor bits and pieces of temporary, homemade magic—are extremely helpful when we have to face some day-to-day phobic situation that is uncomfortably queasy, but still tolerable.

Take a mildly claustrophobic man, for instance, who has to travel by subway now and then. He's aware it makes him nervous to be underground and will go some other route if he can; but if he can't he makes the plunge. Once he's down there, he manages his discomfort by literally rescuing himself from one subway station to the next with fantasy. He holds his breath, closes his eyes, and concentrates on making believe that he's driving the train himself, masterfully overcoming all dangers until he's finally at his stop, whereupon he gets out and abandons the other passengers to their fate without a backward glance or a second thought.

Another kind of rescue fantasy is simply to pretend that the birds you're so terrified of do not exist. "There are no pigeons on the grass, alas," you say over and over to yourself as you walk past a flock of beady-eyed pouters. One woman who is made somewhat uneasy by being in a boat is able to keep her anxiety under control by telling herself firmly that there is nothing under the surface of the waves except six inches of water—after six inches, it's all solid land.

The main drawback to rescue fantasies is that now and then they slip out of our heads into the real world, which usually means we have to get involved in some kind of embarrassed explanation when other people ask us what the hell we think we're doing. Nobody has to know that you ride around on the subway system pretending you're a motorman, of course, and if you're smart you'll keep it to yourself. But if your rescue fantasy demands some kind of prop, the chances are you'll end up in trouble. Like the acrophobe who found he was able to sit on his second-floor terrace if he wound some string in between the railings that were already there and by so doing persuade himself he would not be able to fall through. If nonphobics would only learn that you cannot cure a phobia by laughing at it, that acrophobe and the rest of us would all be much better off.

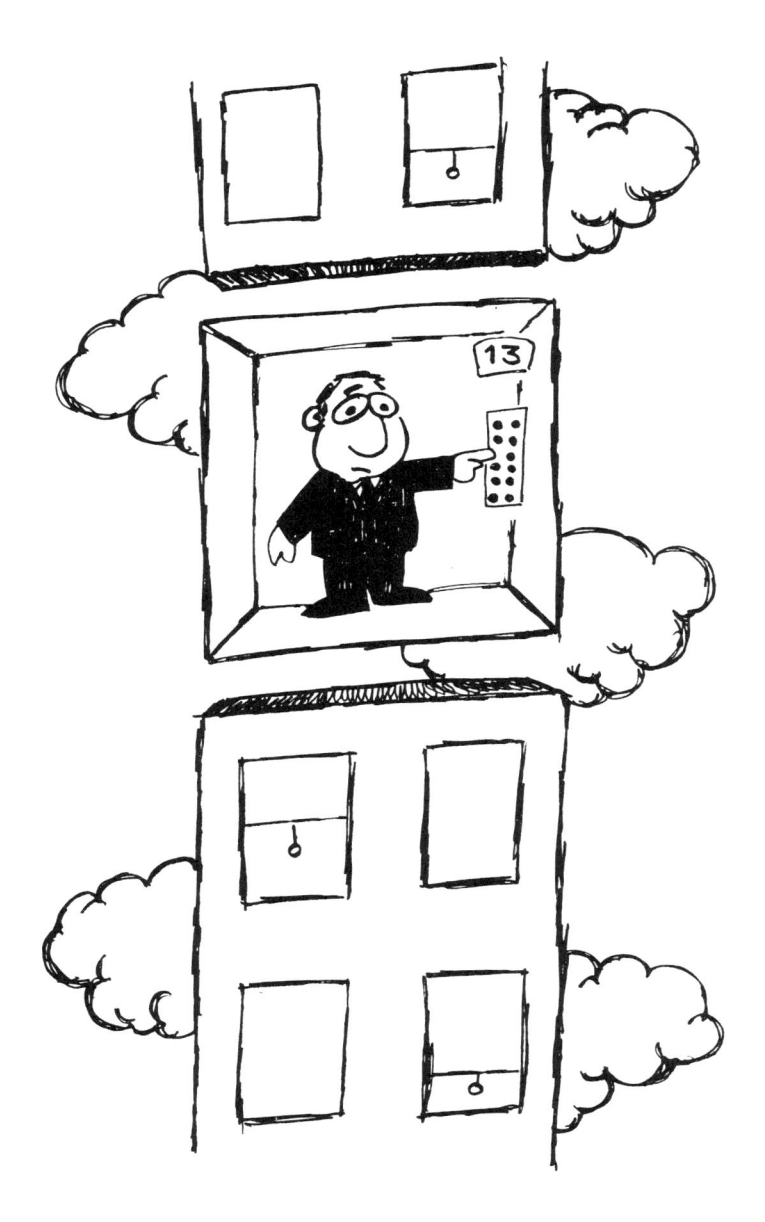

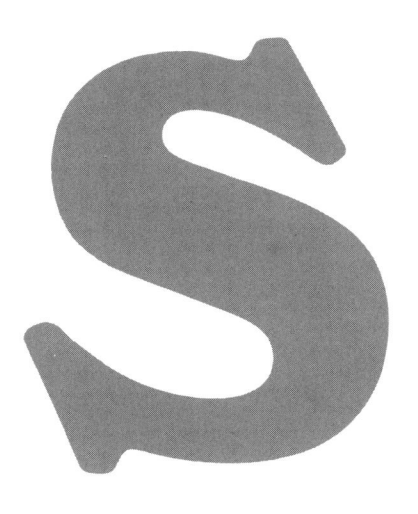

A Caribbean miss named Zenobia
Grew distraught when she thought about obeah.
Voodoo drumbeats at night
Filled her heart with such fright
That "Who goes there," she'd scream, "friend or phobia?"

SUPERSTITION

When the members of a society agree that an idea, object, or situation will commonly be regarded as a symbol *(which see)* as well as a reality, it's called superstition. Those superstitions that involve projected malevolence—the agreed-upon omens of evil—are cultural equivalents of phobia, and the omens themselves amount to communal phobic objects.

Like phobias, superstitions allow us to deal with (that is,

deny) anxiety-provoking hostility by avoiding the symbolic objects that have been picked to serve as displacements. When we don't avoid them (whether or not we think we believe in them), just as when we don't avoid our personal phobic objects, we feel nervously uncomfortable. For those of us who prefer counterphobic behavior to avoidance, superstition also provides for embracing our hostility through a belief in black magic. Most of us stick to avoidance, though—it's at least legal.

It's probably less disturbing to violate a superstition than it is a phobia, but the same reaction is there in both cases. Which of us who, as a child, defiantly stepped on a sidewalk crack with both feet while chanting that frankly murderous formula we all learned by heart the first time we heard it didn't also feel some twinge of uneasiness about the possible consequences? You never can tell. It could be true. And even if it's not, it doesn't hurt to go along—there may be something in it. So would you mind just throwing a pinch of that spilled salt over your shoulder? No, no—the *left* shoulder. Thanks.

All things considered, it's undoubtedly less trouble to be superstitious than phobic, for the same reason that it's easier to make believe in astrology than to depend on your own sense of identity for your character traits: the really tough decisions have already been made in front for you by somebody else, and everybody knows what they are. Unlike the phobic who has to make elaborate explanations to himself and everyone else about why he's terrified of flying, a superstitious person knows that other people already understand and condone his behavior when he walks around ladders, wears a copper bracelet for arthritis, and avoids black cats. He also knows that even if they laugh at him, the chances are they do the same things themselves when they think nobody's looking.

S

Another advantage of this community-approved displacement is that society can pick and choose its omens of evil so they're neither plentiful nor inconvenient. Public opinion is notoriously cautious and conservative, anyway, and hates to offend any large voting bloc. Consequently, the committees on bad omens generally tend to come up with such esoteric things to avoid as three ravens flying due south in a row on a Wednesday, or any old woman living in a hut that whirls through the forest on gigantic chicken feet. You're really going to have to worry a lot about whether or not you'll run into her, right?

Furthermore, if conditions change so that a particular bad omen becomes inconveniently frequent, society simply erases its symbolic value by common consent. When the elevator was invented thirteen was considered a very unlucky number, and for a while everybody pretended together that all tall buildings didn't have a thirteenth floor. But as soon as there were a lot of tall buildings, and it got to be too much trouble to remember to skip from *12* to *14* on the floor numbers, society stopped thinking that thirteen meant anything special, and that was that. This is called progress, and you better believe that for efficiency it sure as hell beats the five years of analysis it can take to get rid of a phobia.

SLEEP PHOBIA

A morbid dread of falling asleep, which is apparently less a fear of sleep itself than of what happens during sleep—that is, dreaming.

As we all know, dreaming gives us the delightful opportunity to do exactly what we please, usually for the first and only time that day. There are some who cannot stand too

S

much of a good thing, though, and faced with the unlimited magical freedom of dreams, these people panic because they're doing and having all those forbidden things.

Children are prone to transient sleep phobias, which may appear after they've had a bad nightmare and disappear after a period of untroubled slumber, just the way behavior theory says they should. Many adults also suffer from sleep phobias in varying degrees of severity and exhaustion.

It's not easy to decide how to deal with a sleep phobia. If you use avoidance, you're dead the next day. If you resort to counterphobic measures and sleep, perchance to dream as much as possible, you miss a lot of meals and eventually might even starve to death. The only thing worse than having a sleep phobia yourself is to be married to somebody who has one and gets lonesome sitting up all night by himself.

SPACE PHOBIA

Space phobias. See Acrophobia, Agoraphobia, *and* Claustrophobia.

SYMBOL

A symbol is anything used by humans to represent, stand for, or disguise thoughts and/or emotions. "Any" thing means just that—animal, vegetable, mineral, abstract, concrete, live, inanimate, man-made, or natural. The thought or emotion being symbolized can also be anything: good, bad, indifferent, simple, complex, beneficial, or malevolent. The

S

symbol itself may be community property, like the flag, or remain a purely private enterprise, like Citizen Kane's Rosebud.

A symbol is as-if magic: people make believe it truly is the thing it stands for. First having made an idol and decided that it will represent holiness, they proceed to fall down and worship it as if it actually were a god. There's no point in trying to argue them out of it, either. You can't beat magic with reason.

All humans symbolize. It's how our heads work. We communicate with each other in the real world using the written and oral symbols of language. We talk to ourselves—and especially the most primitive, least logical, and wholly stubborn parts of our selves—through the dreams, images, and wordless thoughts that make up the language of that world between our ears. We derive many of these personal symbols from our outer life, so that to some extent other people can guess what they mean; but many of them have unique meanings that only we understand. And sometimes we aren't too clear about exactly what's going on, either. Which brings us to phobia.

According to psychoanalytic theory (behaviorists usually don't mention this much, if at all) your phobic object is a symbol that represents (although only to you) an unconscious idea or wish that is unacceptable and hence anxiety-provoking to your conscious mind. Since it makes you too uneasy to experience it directly, you get it out of your head and, you hope, off your hands by finding some symbol for it. Unfortunately, and it does seem rather unfairly, you can't separate what makes you anxious from the anxiety itself, so whatever you use for a symbol will automatically stand for both to your unconscious.

Take Little Hans *(whom see),* for instance. He couldn't admit to himself that he hated his father, so he displaced this unacceptable idea, plus its anxiety, onto horses. He picked horses on the same basis others of us displace onto snakes, insects, fire, dolls, or dogs—they were convenient and conventionally there when he needed something, and because of some personal set of associations, they *looked* right to him. From then on he reacted toward horses with the usual as-if magical thinking. Whenever he saw one, to him it was as if he were seeing both his own hatred and his own guilty anxiety furiously galloping straight toward him on hooves of steel. No wonder he ran. And that running from anxiety is what phobia's all about.